Loving Myself Again

Self-care from A-Z after a NICU stay

Leanne Rose Dorish

Copyright © 2020, Leanne Rose Dorish

All rights reserved. No part of this publication may be reproduced, distributed or transmitted in any form or by any means, including photocopying, recording or other electronic or mechanical methods, without the prior written permission of the publisher, except in the case of brief quotations embodied in reviews and certain other non-commercial uses permitted by copyright law.

ISBN: 978-1-7772088-0-6

Book Cover design by: rebecacovers
Cover image credit: Olga Yakovenko
Edited by: Danielle Steiner-Janzen

ACCESS MY SELF-CARE START-UP VIDEO FOR FREE!

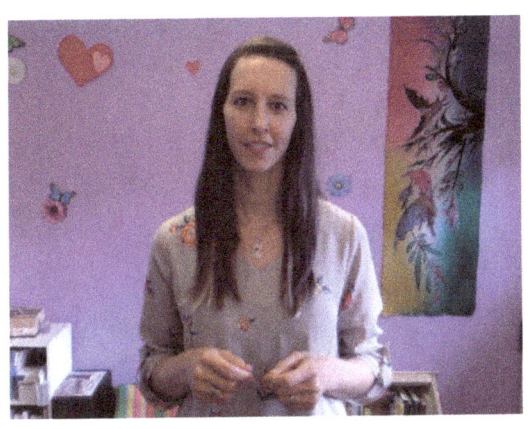

READ THIS FIRST

Success comes from starting something new. I walk you through the steps you need in order to start your self-care routine and keep it.

As a thank you for buying my book, I'd like to give you access to my Self-Care Start-Up Video 100% FREE!

Go to

www.mynicufamily.com/LMAfreegifts

Dedication

This book is dedicated to my incredibly patient and supportive husband, Scott. Thank you for continuously believing in me.

With Love Always,

Your Leannie

"Magical moments come out by shifting perspective."

~Leanne Rose Dorish

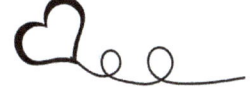

Contents

Introduction

How to Use This Book

A is for Attention
B is for Bonding
C is for Creativity
D is for Downtime
E is for Empathy
F is for Friends
G is for Gratitude
H is for Honour
I is for Intuition
J is for Juiciness
K is for Kindness
L is for Love
M is for Movement
N is for Nurturing
O is for Observation
P is for Patience
Q is for Quiet
R is for Rest

S is for Spirit
T is for Time
U is for Understanding
V is for Voice
W is for Work
X is for Xenialness
Y is for You
Z is for Zest

Acknowledgements
About The Author

Introduction

Whether your child was in a Neonatal Intensive Care Unit (NICU) or Special Care Nursery (SCN) for one day, one year or somewhere in between, it is usually not where you expected to be. Wearing a hospital gown (and maybe even gloves) to reach through two small windows of a plexiglass wall into the world of your newborn child can bring so many questions and emotions.

Taking care of yourself during this time is a journey of struggles and triumphs—a journey that continuously needs to be refocused and approached from new perspectives.

My son, Skye, arrived nine weeks early and spent two months in the NICU. When I was first home with Skye, I was lost. I hadn't connected my overwhelming emotions with the traumas we had gone through. Even when I finally did recognize that I was experiencing post-traumatic stress symptoms, I did not want to go to counselling. Let's face it: being a trauma counsellor myself, I knew that working through emotions from trauma is a lot of work. I had a brand-new baby home from the hospital with a compromised immune system, so I did not want to go out—all I wanted to do was sleep. But I finally did pick myself up and start going to a counsellor, which was a saving grace. I realized how much of myself I had forgotten. Skye needed so much of me and because I wanted to protect him, I had stopped thinking about myself. The depletion showed.

My health became an issue, somewhat due to the traumatic birth and the two months in the NICU not taking care of myself and also due to feeling trapped in this new life of chaos. My body did not like the stress of needing to keep appointments or of driving in a big city. Internally, my body had shown me signs of stress, and now externally, it was telling me something needed to change, or else.

This book is an easy read for the busy parent after coming home with a baby from the NICU. It could also be used for anyone who feels busyness has taken over their life. It is a general go-to when you are in need of a self-care idea. My practices are not the conventional suggestions you see in the self-help book section: the ideas in this book come straight from my heart and personal experience as a trauma counsellor and NICU graduate mama.

Every chapter is written with compassion for you—who is exhausted, who has too many NICU follow-up appointments, or who feels there isn't enough time to invest in self-care (or all of the above!).

How to Use This Book

There are many ways you can use this book and start practicing the ideas in each chapter. One day you may want to start at the beginning of the alphabet; the next day you might go to the first letter of your name. Or you may just want to randomly open the book and see what letter you land on.

Regardless of the order, you can practice each of these ideas for a day or a week—the fun part is, it's up to you! Be conscious of wanting to start new habits. Frequently retrace your steps to see which habits were easy to implement and which ones still need some work.

There are a few ways to improve your self-care practice:

- Write the idea you are practicing on a note card and put it on your fridge or in your pocket for easy, quick reference.

- Write one key word on the bathroom mirror with soap as a reminder.

- Create a wallpaper screen for your computer and/or phone with a caring word or phrase on it.

- Use the affirmations from each chapter as mantras.

With this book, you will start taking care of yourself in new ways so you don't become bored, frustrated or "clichéd out" from regular practices.

You are an amazing person, and you are giving so much of yourself to others. You deserve to create a more mindful and conscious way of living with yourself now that you are home from the NICU.

A is for Attention

Most of your Attention is probably going to the child you are caring for. The next person who receives your Attention could be your partner or maybe an ailing parent. Third on the Attention list might be the family pet...do you see where I'm going here? We are spread thin even when it comes to just regular life responsibilities, and as a NICU parent finally at home with our baby, we can easily find ourselves falling farther down that rabbit hole.

Where are you on this Attention list?

Giving Attention to yourself at least a few times a week might seem totally out of the question. You might be thinking, "I'm lucky if I can find time for myself once a year!"

When you give so much of yourself to help your family or those around you, it can be easy to forget about your own needs and well-being.

I was so focused on Skye when he was first in the NICU that I would literally forget to eat. No joke. We couldn't bring food next to the incubators, so I just wouldn't eat—because as you know, you want to spend every possible millisecond with that baby in the isolette. My husband had to frequently hound me to go and eat something. I learned my lesson the hard way, because I ended up getting very sick.

Attention to yourself is so, so, SO important, especially if you are responsible for helping someone else. In order to help others and be a good role model to those who depend on you, you need to practice taking care of yourself the same way you take care of others.

Over the past few years, I have discovered two simple ways of prioritizing some Attention for myself:

1) I set an alarm on my phone with a message that might say something like, "Give yourself some Attention right now," or "I see you! Take a big belly breath!" I then take as much time as I can in that moment just to look inward. Sometimes it's one second for a breath, and sometimes I can fit in two to five minutes of reflection.

2) I have accountability partners. Whether it's a friend who will text me, my husband at home to check in or an online friend available for messaging, I get that reminder to take a moment for myself. I sometimes have a two-minute date with that person where we chat about the day and send each other some gratitude. It's a wonderful way to create space for myself and feel supported at the same time.

When you choose to be good to yourself, it's a lot easier to be good to those around you.

Affirmation: I am allowed to give Attention to myself.

B is for Bonding

Taking time to Bond with yourself might sound a bit weird, and yet when you find time to get to know yourself again, you can help those around you know you better too.

Another way to look at Bonding with yourself is to Bond with your baby or with your partner. This is an important part of self-care. Safe relationships provide a place to be yourself and create healthy habits. This is extremely important when you have gone through a difficult situation in your life, like having had a baby in the NICU or SCN.

Bonding with someone on an emotional level creates space to exchange ideas and provide new perspectives on old habits.

There are two particular ways I Bond with myself:

1) When given the opportunity to have a few moments to myself, I will often go into a room and just "be." I put my feelings of guilt that

I'm "not doing something" to the side, and I sit on the floor and absorb my surroundings. I have made my office into my sanctuary now, but in my old house I kept a few things inside my bedroom closet that made me feel safe and able to Bond with myself. Back then, I would open the closet doors, sit on the floor and give myself some time to focus on my own thoughts.

2) I take myself out on dates. You might be thinking I'm totally bizarre—that's okay! But when I can, I will go and have lunch out by myself somewhere I wouldn't normally go. Before Skye came into my life, I even used to go to movies by myself. It gives me strength to know that I can really do anything!

Take some time this week to Bond with yourself or cuddle with someone you love. This Bonding with your child or partner will give you an opportunity to connect with your emotions.

Affirmation: It is okay for me to get to know myself again.

C is for Creativity

Being Creative with the way you live after the NICU can help you feel like yourself again.

Perhaps before the baby arrived you enjoyed painting or baking or gardening, but then you found yourself in the NICU and that Creativity was put on hold. Now that baby is home, it is time to start bringing your interests back.

Here are some ways I have brought Creativity back into my life:

1) I get Skye involved in the Creativity. Let's face it: Skye is with me a lot, and he is usually the reason I can't get my work done. Once I figured out that giving him his own set of paints or a spatula or other "tool" would keep him happily occupied, we were rocking it!

2) We have a colouring book on our kitchen table. When there is a lull in leaving the house, cooking or cleaning, that easily accessible

colouring book is relaxing and fun and gets the creative juices flowing.

Being Creative takes on countless forms when you let yourself feel free again.

Affirmation: It is okay to do things I enjoy.

D is for Downtime

This is rejuvenation time for you.

When our minds don't have any time to rest (other than sleep), it means we are pushing too hard and can become cranky, bossy, obsessive and all sorts of other not-so-fun attitudes.

While Downtime may seem similar to the section on Attention a few chapters back, I see Downtime as time when you don't have to be "on" or answering to someone else. It is a moment or two when you can create a peaceful space for yourself.

These are two quick things I do to ensure I get a little Downtime:

1) I put a book in the bathroom—a book that I actually want to read, not one that I have to read. And we all know that the bathroom is the only place where we can get one minute to ourselves (...maybe).

E is for Empathy

Looking inside yourself to take a break from the constant bombardment of "coulda-woulda-shoulda" will create space to fill with love.

Pay attention to how you talk to yourself or about yourself. This is an important part of having Empathy. You can become your own worst enemy by saying negative things about yourself. Your self-talk is sometimes worse than how you talk about others.

Being compassionate and Empathetic with yourself will improve the ways you can be kind to those around you.

Here are two ways you can find more Empathy for yourself:

1) Remember that you are human too. Even though others might see you as this "can-do-everything" or "totally with-it" person, you can have too many expectations on yourself. Remember to draw the line somewhere.

2) I stay up just ten minutes later than everyone else. I find it very peaceful when the house is quiet and the lights are low. Even if I am totally exhausted, I will get some me-time and be able to just slow down. This can also help me sleep better at night.

As a caregiver, it is important to give yourself moments during the week to relax your shoulders and let your mind be free.

Affirmation: I am allowed to have time to myself.

2) Instead of telling yourself, "I should have done X," take a step back and put yourself in your own shoes. This might sound funny, but we can lose perspective on our own lives when we compare ourselves to others. Try rephrasing your words into non-comparing ones: for example, "The next time I do X, I'm going to change Y about it."

In finding Empathy for your own life, you will bring compassion and Empathy into your routines. This will reduce your stress, calm your nerves and keep you focused on what is most important to you.

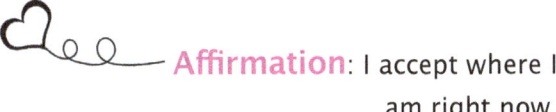

Affirmation: I accept where I am right now.

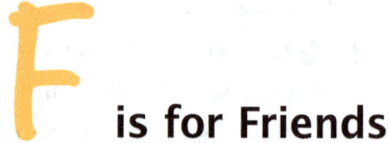 **is for Friends**

Interaction with Friends, whether they're close or far away, is an important part of self-care.

Friends can be people you have had in your life for a long time or someone you just found last week. They can be your parents, your partner or even your pets. They are souls that you feel comfortable sharing yourself with.

Giving yourself time with a Friend can bring new energy.

Here are two ways I connect with Friends:

1) I talk to them on the phone, so I can hear their tone of voice and envision their face. This brings me the energy of that person who cares for me and uplifts my spirit. You can also have a video call for the same reasons.

2) I write postcards to Friends. I know it's considered "old-school" now, but buying a postcard and writing a quick note to a Friend can brighten my day—and theirs. My girlfriend

in Germany and I rarely email or text, opting instead to write letters and send cards. It somehow seems to bring more sunshine!

Be creative with how you connect with Friends. Allow them to be a part of the chaos that you think no one understands. If they are a NICU parent like yourself, then that chaos won't seem crazy to them at all.

Affirmation: My Friends are my allies; I can let them support me.

G is for Gratitude

Use words of thanks for things you already have in your life and things you would like to see in your future.

Being Grateful for something in the future may seem strange. However, the angels, the universe and even your very own molecules will hear what you are looking for and be able to answer you with what is meant to be.

Here are some ways I use Gratitude on a daily basis:

1) When faced with a difficult situation, I project my Gratitude for a peaceful and safe outcome. For example, before I cross the highway at a difficult intersection I say, "Thank you, angels, for helping us to safely cross the highway today."

2) I start the day with saying out loud what I feel Grateful for. Skye will even chime in with things he enjoys. Sometimes it's Lego, sometimes it's diggers—and other times, he will get very deep

and be Grateful for the people in his life that have touched his heart.

Gratitude is a key piece to thriving mental wellness.

Affirmation: I can be Grateful for this moment.

H is for Honour

Respecting the events and situations that are happening to us and around us is not always easy. Honouring a frustrating issue takes courage, patience and practice.

Allow yourself to Honour your own actions and decisions, even if you would do something differently next time. Understanding that you did what you could with the knowledge you had will help you in future situations.

There are two ways that I practice using Honour in my life:

1) I recognize all of the powerful decisions I have made: looking for alternative health care for my family, helping Skye thrive with his diagnoses and learning to share my experiences with others.

2) I respect that I don't always have control. Not being in control is a big issue for me, and it

has been difficult to recognize that there are other people and powers at play. Honouring that understanding has allowed me to step back and release some of my frustrations.

Accepting certain situations is not easy, and if you want to move away from the pain of a difficult circumstance, reframe it with what was Honourable in the moment.

Affirmation: I accept my actions and learn from the past.

I is for Intuition

Intuition is instinctive. When we "just know" something, this is our Intuition coming through to guide us.

As a NICU parent, I have learned to tap into this deep Intuition when it comes to making decisions for Skye. It takes practice and awareness to learn to listen to it and once you start to see how your instincts make life easier, there is no going back. Learning to trust your Intuition will help you feel confident with your decisions.

I practice listening to my Intuition in these two ways:

1) When an idea just will not leave me alone, I have learned to stop and listen. I often get the same thoughts, images or words repeated in my head, and I have discovered that this is my deep Intuition telling me to move forward with this part of my life.

2) I meditate. I know it's probably cliché to say that now, but it honestly works. Whether I

get a five-minute block of time to sit or a few moments to zone out as I do the dishes, it all counts.

We don't get enough quiet time, so create some for yourself and tap into that fabulous Intuition.

Affirmation: I can learn to trust my Intuition.

J is for Juiciness

Mmm...this one is fun!

When I think of self-care being Juicy, I think of my life as being full of awesomeness. Whether it's laughing, prioritizing "me" time or playing trucks with Skye, abundance can come in so many forms.

To some, a Juicy life might mean too much gossip or drama, which is not what NICU parents need. Instead, think of Juiciness as all the fun stuff you can bring into your (and your family's) life.

There are lots of ways to have a Juicy life, but there are two particular ways I input Juiciness into my life:

1) I remember to fill my cup as well as my family's. I have some hobbies that my husband or son don't find interesting, so I take time to have fun doing those things all on my own. And if Skye does become interested (like when I was doing a little sewing project and he wanted to

know what I was up to), I include him and we share the fun.

2) I try new things—even as simple as walking a new trail or finding a new way to play in my existing space. (There are always new ways a couch-cushion fort can be constructed!)

Find different ways to bring awesomeness into your life so that it feels Juicy and full of new experiences.

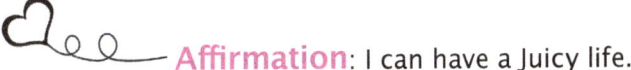 **Affirmation**: I can have a Juicy life.

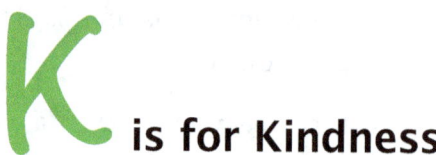 is for Kindness

Being Kind brings you to a different level of understanding yourself and others. I think of Kindness as a personal goal that turns into an outward blessing.

Begin by looking at how Kind you are to yourself: Do you say nasty things about yourself in your head? Do you make fun of yourself in front of others? When did you last look in the mirror and tell yourself that you are beautiful?

Kindness starts within. It has to start with you so you can be a role model without even knowing it. Live in Kindness and others will follow your example.

These are a couple ways I practice Kindness:

1) When I'm cranky, I take a moment to ask myself why I'm upset. I give myself a little counselling session in order to have space to be heard and cared for. This is me being Kind to myself so I can be Kind to others.

2) I watch what I say about myself both in my head and when talking to others. Jokingly saying, "Oh yeah, I'm so stupid sometimes!" is actually being quite mean. I would never, ever say this about anyone else, so why would I say this about myself?

Kindness starts with you.

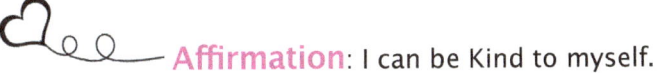 **Affirmation**: I can be Kind to myself.

L is for Love

Love can have a different meaning to everyone, but ultimately it is personal, enveloping and unconditional.

We often forget that we can lead with Love in everything we say and do, when we live in a society that does not generally lead with Love.

Here are two ways I create Love in my daily life:

1) I feel it in my body when I use the word "Love." Instead of just casually saying, "Love you!" to someone, I feel it in my bones. I let the word exude its meaning from my whole self and hope the other person can feel the energy of my Love.

2) Forgiveness. If I have done something wrong or if someone else has acted against me, I work on forgiving myself first. This might have to be done with the help of a counsellor or therapist, depending on how deep the situation is. Love comes from understanding a situation and

allowing for forgiveness, even in the smallest of ways.

Recognizing that Love is a powerful tool can give you new opportunities and a lighter heart.

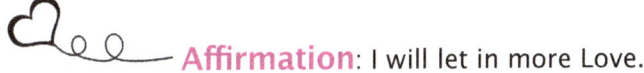 **Affirmation**: I will let in more Love.

M is for Movement

Your body will thank you if you Move more often.

Sometimes it is as simple as standing up and getting a few stretches in before having to sit down again. If you remember to take care of yourself even a fraction of the time that you take care of your family, you will notice a difference in your tolerance levels, mental health and physical capabilities.

There are many ways you can Move in your daily life, but here are two ways I incorporate Movement into my life:

1) I walk where I can. For example, I will find a distant parking spot at the grocery store so I can get a few more footsteps in. Or I will get off the bus one or two stops before my planned stop.

2) Skye and I (and Scott when he's home) have spontaneous dance parties. These are so much fun! I can see how my little Skye is growing in

his motor abilities, whether we're dancing on our feet or just Moving our arms. We also try out new Moves, and a lot of the time it turns into a sort of physiotherapy session without Skye knowing. (Tee-hee-hee...)

Movement is so very important for your physical, mental, emotional, spiritual and social self.

Affirmation: I can Move more frequently.

N is for Nurturing

When you think of being Nurtured, what comes to mind? Perhaps a warm hug, a compassionate note, an understanding teacher? We often think of our childhood or how we treat our own children when we think of being Nurtured.

Did you know you can Nurture yourself, even in adulthood?

You can train your mind and body to feel Nurtured even when there is no one else doing the Nurturing. Nurture yourself with kindness and quiet moments.

There are two primary ways I Nurture myself:

1) I make sure I have healthy food every day. Even when I am travelling or super busy, I seek out food that will nourish and Nurture my body and mind.

2) I create space to inspire my mind and Nurture my soul. I love to learn about new things, so I

consistently take time to either read, watch or listen to something that is new to me.

Even giving yourself one of those funny and slightly awkward self-hugs can be a way to show yourself a bit of Nurturing.

Affirmation: It is okay for me to feel Nurtured.

O is for Observation

Observing yourself gives room for growth.

When you can take the time to Observe how you are currently living or how you handled a past situation, you can learn what you would like to do similarly or differently in the future.

Observation also finds ways to show us how not to be. I'm sure you have watched someone else react poorly to a situation and thought, "I don't want to be like that."

Here are a couple ways I Observe in my life:

1) I take time to reflect. If I have a lasting feeling about something that happened during my day, especially if it's a negative feeling, I take time to think about it. Sometimes it's hard because I feel guilty or ashamed of my behaviour, but more often I can find the glimmer of guidance in it and work with that.

2) In a frustrating moment involving others, I do my best to Observe what the other person might be feeling or trying to say. If I'm frustrated, then the other person probably is too. I give my very best self in order to be kind to my frustration, and then kindness can be given to both parties involved.

Practice Observing yourself. It is not an easy task, but the resulting understanding and insight can be rewarding.

Affirmation: I give myself permission to be an Observer.

p is for Patience

Patience is not something we are generally taught in an easy way. We're told to "be Patient," or "just wait a second" (which is never actually one second). We have to figure out what Patience looks like for that other person in order to seem like we have Patience.

As we become familiar with how our kids can push our boundaries, we learn how to have a relationship with Patience itself.

I have found the following to be effective ways to practice Patience:

1) When we should have been out the door X minutes ago but Skye is taking his sweet time, I can catch myself feeling frustrated. So I take a breath and tell myself, "Being Patient right now is easier than us getting mad at each other and slowing the process down even more!"

2) I have Patience with myself when I'm procrastinating. If I try to push myself to

work on a particular project when I'm not in the mood, I generally don't have a good time finishing it. I might get angry or be unhappy with the end result. But when I'm in the right mood to finish the task, the answers come easily, and the project is often completed in half the time.

Patience takes practice. Catching yourself in the impatience is the first step.

Affirmation: I can practice Patience for both myself and others.

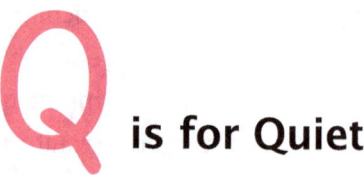 is for Quiet

Quiet can be the silence from the world around you, but it can also be the calm from within you.

Self-care is all about tapping into your voice and your needs in order to survive and thrive in your everyday life. In order to figure out what those needs are, you often need Quiet.

Meditation is a popular way to find some Quiet in your life, but it's not always the easiest way.

So, here are two ways I find Quiet in my day:

1) I close my eyes. It's amazing what this does for me. When I close my eyes, my shoulders relax, my mind wanders and things around me seem to just "be." By closing my eyes, even if only for a moment, I am creating a block for one of my senses, which helps remove some distractions and allow for more Quiet.

2) I notice the Quiet right after everyone has fallen asleep. The house is mostly silent: there

are no voices, there are no extra noises coming from outside. I often find myself staying up just a few extra minutes to enjoy the Quiet.

Learn to find Quiet within you even when there is noise around you. Those few seconds can rejuvenate you for the rest of the day.

Affirmation: I give myself permission to find Quiet.

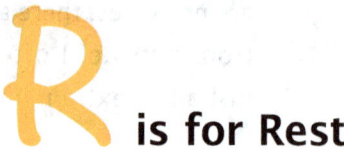 is for Rest

You can relax and take it easy, but to Rest is to let yourself feel looked after and restored.

Giving yourself time to relax probably doesn't happen a lot. You might even wait until you get sick to really Rest (and even then, sometimes you just don't have time).

Here are two ways I Rest on a regular basis:

1) The shower is a great place to feel rejuvenated. Even though a shower's purpose is to clean, you can find Rest in slowing down and enjoying a quiet moment in the shower.

2) I put my feet up. I know this probably seems obvious to mention, and yet when I put my feet up on the footstool my body knows I'm Resting. I breathe more from my belly and my shoulders are able to release some tension.

Rest and relaxation can come in small moments here and there, or you can choose to take a bigger chunk of time away from it all. However you choose to make your life a bit more Restful, your body and mind will be thankful.

Affirmation: I am allowed to Rest.

S is for Spirit

I see the concept of Spirit in two ways: one is for the Spirit within us that is connected to the higher powers, and the other is the Spirit that comes out when we cheer ourselves on and find the strength to keep going.

Ultimately, these could be the same thing. To start a self-care journey, it can be easier to think of them as separate.

These are of couple examples of how I have Spirit in my daily life:

1) I often do a little dance in the kitchen so my cheerleader-from-within can keep me going and give me energy and strength.

2) I connect with my higher power through practicing meditation, doing yoga, reading, going for a walk outdoors or just sitting and looking out the window. I reconnect with the mind within me that has roots in this earth and thoughts in the stars.

Whether you identify as being a Spiritual person or you just enjoy a good walk in nature, getting energy from other sources can be helpful when you feel stuck or gloomy.

Affirmation: I have a Spirit within to help me.

T is for Time

It often gives me a headache or overwhelms me when I think of doing everything I need to get done. And then I don't want to do any of it. Sound familiar?

So, I break things down into doable snippets and tell myself, "I have Time."

Here are two ways I use Time to benefit me regularly:

1) I use timers. Instead of sitting in front of my to-do list, I put on a timer and give myself one task. Regardless of how long I think it's going to take, that timer gets me started; then I either don't stop because I'm on a roll, or if I have to stop, I know exactly where to pick up next Time.

2) Instead of worrying about how much Time I have let pass, I look at how much Time I have ahead of me. This is a total willingness to change perspective. I'm still human and torment myself often for wasted Time. But it

helps immensely when I can shift my thinking into looking ahead.

Let Time be a useful tool instead of a pressure.

Affirmation: Time is on my side; I have Time.

U is for Understanding

We generally have more compassion and Understanding for other people than we do for ourselves.

When I am upset or annoyed, I allow myself to feel those feelings. When another person is involved in the emotions, I do my best to Understand my thoughts before connecting with the other person. Finding compassion for my own feelings helps me work through difficult situations.

Here's how I use Understanding in my life:

1) When I get upset with Skye and feel badly afterwards, I often have to put myself aside first in order to tend to him. In minding his feelings, I am showing Understanding for my own actions and reactions. I apologize for my part of the situation. Then, when I have time, I figure out what I would do differently next time.

2) I sometimes have fears others around me don't Understand. As the mother of a NICU graduate, my worries might seem more far-fetched than those of the other moms around me. And when I feel this way and wonder if I should change my mind, I remember where I've come from. No one else has walked this walk, and I can Understand why I'm fearing what I am.

In both of the above situations, my Understanding does not present itself the same way every time. It takes a lot of practice and self-talk to figure out where I can give myself compassion and where I need to grow as an individual.

Affirmation: I can learn to Understand myself better.

V is for Voice

When you hear the word "Vocalize," you might think of yelling or singing or anything that involves getting louder than your regular Voice volume. But using your Voice means that you can communicate in multiple ways.

As a NICU parent, you might sometimes think that you shouldn't speak up. You might think there are other fights to fight or that others should speak before you. But you deserve to be heard and cared for. By using your Voice, you can help yourself and those around you.

There are two primary ways I use my Voice:

1) When my emotions are high, I take the time to ground myself. Then, in a gentle way, I let my husband know what I'm thinking. Sometimes my body tells the story before I use words, but at least it's not being bottled up inside me.

2) I sing. I sometimes sing out my emotions or my thoughts. Other times I sing to Skye in bed. It shifts the energy within me because it expresses something for me. Even if you don't think you can sing, expressing your thoughts through song can provide release.

Share your ideas through Vocalizing. It is a good way to learn more about yourself.

Affirmation: My Voice is a beautiful tool.

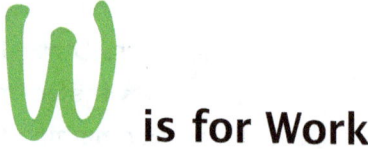 is for Work

When I was first home after the NICU, I found myself going stir-crazy, because I was used to Working and having time to myself. Instead of viewing Work as something that takes us away from our babies and all the other necessary chores at home, look at how it creates space for you to be a different you—whether you Work at home or outside the home.

Here is how I implement Work into my life:

1) I am physically away from the house with some of my clients, and this gives me some time to be a different me. I find that when I'm productive and have a little bit of time away, I can be a better mom and partner.

2) Work is something I play with at home. It's a practicing of habits that helps make my NICU Work more effective, whether it's when I'm giving a seminar or talking with a client. For example, Skye, Scott and I will all do voice exercises together. Sometimes they will just

listen as I do them in the kitchen, but whichever way we do it, it turns into family fun!

However you view Work, look at how it makes you feel. If you can't find anything enjoyable about the Work you do, perhaps it's time to shift to something new.

Affirmation: My Work is important.

X is for Xenialness

To be Xenial means to be friendly or hospitable. We need to remember to be Xenial to ourselves more often.

Here are two ways I implement Xenialness in my daily life:

1) I cut myself slack when I do something that is lousy or silly in hindsight. I would give my friend a break, so why not be friendly to myself?

2) When life gets too busy, I play with Skye. When I'm busy with work or chores, this is often the time he taps into that pressure and wants me to play with him even more. When I see how busy I have become, I disconnect from those tasks and do crafts or play diggers with Skye for a while. It shifts my energy and puts me in a better headspace.

Being Xenial with myself allows me to be friendlier to everyone in my life and feel better about my tasks.

Affirmation: I am friendly to myself so I can be friendlier to others.

Y is for You

You are the best gauge for what You need. How often do You listen to Yourself? How often do You put Yourself first? Likely not as often as You would like.

There are lots of ways to prioritize Yourself, but here are two methods I use to put more of You (or me) into daily life:

1) I continuously reconnect with myself through my thoughts. If I'm getting worked up, I take a moment and really look at what's happening around me. Then I go within to see what my inner needs are. This takes less than a second once You have practiced and become familiar with the process.

2) I make sure I eat properly. This might seem trivial, but it's a big deal for me. If I'm not eating because I think I'm too busy, or I'm not eating healthy options for my body, I can get cranky with myself and with others. No one—

not even me—wants to see that Leanne very often!

Taking care of You means that your children and family get the best You possible. The constant bombardment of parenting a NICU graduate seems endless until You focus on Yourself for a moment. The attention on Yourself opens up the real You.

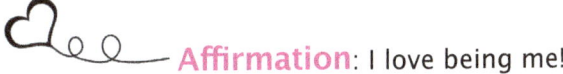 **Affirmation**: I love being me!

Z is for Zest

Zest means to have great enthusiasm and energy. It is a feeling of vitality for life and brings hope, fun and excitement.

Having Zest in your life helps you learn more about who you are now and helps provide a sense of liveliness in your daily life.

Here are two ways I have Zest in my daily existence:

1) I look around and remind myself that life is only as exciting as I make it. It's on me to consciously choose to have a hopeful outlook on life. So, I'll put on some funky old music, and Skye and I will bust a move, even if it's just while we are cleaning up toys.

2) When Skye is playing dress-up or being super silly, I recognize that he is full of Zest. This makes me want some of that, so I will ask him to dress me up and we'll be silly together.

Zestful energy can be easier to feel when you have taken care of yourself. When you get enough sleep, eat well and take that extra care, it's much easier to feel Zest for the life you have around you.

However you experience Zest, bringing that energy into your awareness will bring more joy and light to yourself—and the rest of the world.

Affirmation: I am full of Zest!

Acknowledgements

Thank you, Creator, for honouring me with this journey and gifting me the people who have made a difference along the way.

If it were not for the nurses, doctors, specialists and staff at BC Women's Hospital NICU, I would be writing a very different book today. Thank you for all of the time, care and expertise you gave us during our 60-day stay with you.

A special thank-you goes to my incredible Women's Monday Mastermind group (Abigail Joseph, Holli Howard and Shira Coleman) for continuously having faith in my ideas and encouraging me with each step toward fulfilling my dreams.

Thank you to my dear friend Jaclyn Foster, who is both an inspiring accountabilibuddy and incredible author. And to my sweet editor, Danielle, who is a wizardess with words.

A loving thank-you to Mom (Barb) and Dad (Doug) who have both been amazing teachers in my life. How to have love and compassion for others and maintain a strong work ethic are just a few things I have been blessed to learn from you.

An immense sense of gratitude goes to my sweet boy, Skye. Without you, this purpose may never have been realized. You are the stars in my eyes and the song in my heart. Forever and for always, you are my baby.

My deepest and most intense gratitude goes to my husband. Scott, you are the reason I finished writing this book. I have been able to fulfill this dream of becoming a published author because of your support, encouragement and pure, unconditional love. Thank you for taking care of Skye so often. With all of my heart and my spirit, I thank you. Love you always!

About The Author

Love is my first language.

I am the proud mama of a 2014 NICU graduate. As a registered clinical counsellor, my private practice focuses on treating and relieving the symptoms of trauma. Recognizing the trauma that NICU stays can create, I have turned my 11 years of trauma therapy experience into building community and resources for NICU graduate families.

I am an author, speaker and
guest blogger on the topic.
My online resources can be found at
www.mynicufamily.com
and at @my_nicu_family on
Instagram and Facebook.

I live a quiet life in the Southern Interior of British Columbia, Canada, with my husband and son.
I am truly blessed to be surrounded by nature and the wildness of Mother Earth.

www.ingramcontent.com/pod-product-compliance
Lightning Source LLC
Chambersburg PA
CBHW070047120526
44589CB00035B/2432